this publication is strictly prohibited and any storage of this document is not allowed unless with written permission from the publisher. All rights reserved.

The information provided herein is stated to be truthful and consistent, in that any liability, in terms of inattention or otherwise, by any usage or abuse of any policies, processes, or directions contained within is the solitary and utter responsibility of the recipient reader. Under no circumstances will any legal responsibility or blame be held against the publisher for any reparation, damages, or monetary loss due to the information herein, either directly or indirectly.

Respective authors own all copyrights not held by the publisher.

The information herein is offered for informational purposes solely and is universal as so. The presentation of the information is without contract or any type of guarantee assurance.

Table of contents

INTRODUCTION

What is potty?

A potty is a deep bowl which a small child uses instead of a toilet.

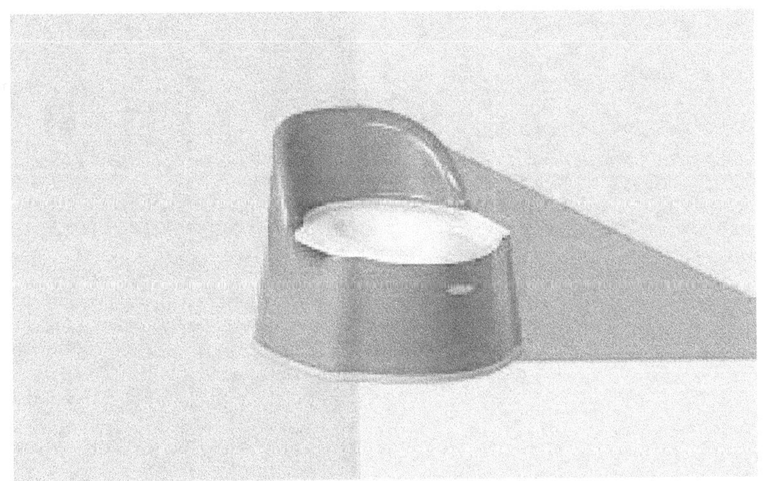

Potty training

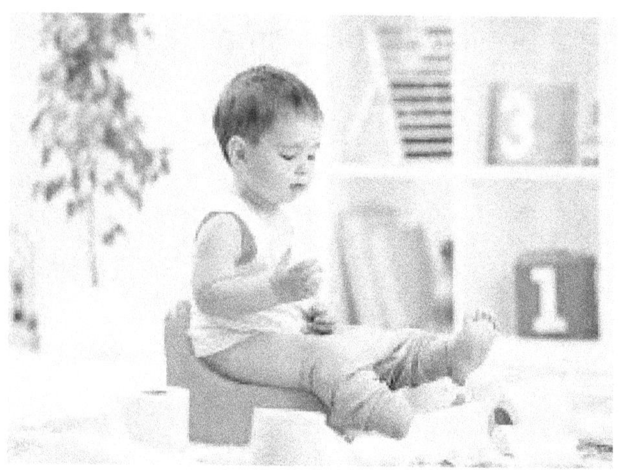

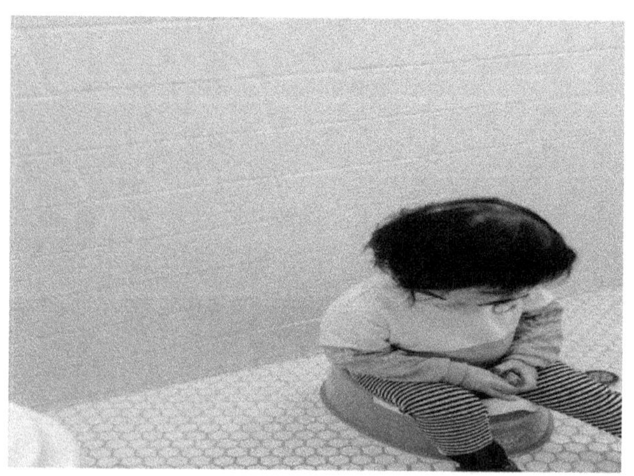

Potty training or toilet training, is a major milestone for toddlers as they learn to listen to their body and use the bathroom to empty their bladder and bowels. It also means no more diaper changes for you. Before you dive into potty training, make sure your toddler is actually ready. It will save both you and your child a lot of frustrations.

Types of potty training

People choose to go about potty training in many different ways. Here is a look at some popular methods:

- **Brazelton Child-Oriented Potty Training**

Supported by the American Academy of Pediatrics, child-oriented potty training is a positive, nonthreatening approach that involves beginning potty training when your child shows signs of readiness (typically after 18 months old).

The idea is for the child to instigate the trips to the bathroom and for the parents to talk about and encourage potty use by using praise, not shame or force. Often, toddlers will continue to wear diapers or pull-ups during the process.

- **Infant Potty Training**

Also known as elimination communication, infant potty training typically begins around 1 to 4 months old and involves rushing the infant to the bathroom when you see certain clues from the baby (such as vocalizations) or patterns based on timing of meals and sleep. Disposable diapers are typically avoided, thought many parents use cloth diapers at night so their baby can feel when they are wet. This method is often messy and may not be the best option for infants who go to daycare or have nannies.

- **Parent-Led Potty Training**

As the name implies, parents take the lead and create a potty break schedule when their toddler shows signs of readiness, taking them to the bathroom every two to three hours during the day. An alternative schedule may involve taking them before and after every meal, between activities, before nap time and bedtime, and upon waking. While parent-led potty training is a good method for toddlers with multiple caregivers, some say it prevents the child from recognizing their own body signs as quickly.

- **3-Day Potty Training**

Popular among parents for its quick results, the 3-day potty training method involves hunkering down at home for—you guessed it—three days and letting your child go diaper-free while you vigilantly take them to the potty. The process can be stressful and accidents will happen, but many children quickly learn to recognize the signs that they need to go and are able to successfully get themselves to the potty on time.

When to start potty training

Many parents choose to potty train a child at a specific age, such as 18 months or 2 years old, but that strategy can backfire if a child is not ready. How old is old enough to potty train? Like most things with kids, it depends.

Parents may have heard stories about a potty-trained 2-month-old, but many children aren't ready until after their second birthday. Some toddlers may not be ready for the potty until they are approaching age 3—and that is okay.

If they are not interested yet, do not force it. Chances are their interest will be piqued sooner rather than later.

Signs your child is ready for potty training

One way to tell if your child is ready is if they have reached certain developmental milestones. For example, potty training is often more successful if your toddler can walk and run, communicate, follow directions (for example, find the bathroom, turn on the light, pull down pants and underwear, and wash their hands), and has strong enough muscles to get on and off of the potty.

Your child must also be mentally ready, which is why it is important to avoid potty training during potentially stressful times, including the transition from a crib to a bed, holidays, vacations, having a new baby in the house, divorce, or moving to a new home.

Other signs that indicate your child is ready for potty training include:

• Shows interest in what you are doing when you go to the bathroom

• Has an interest in keeping clean or dry

• Recognizes when they are in the process of going (hides behind furniture or curtains, or goes to another room to pee or poop)

• Expresses a desire to use the potty

• Shows independence, saying things like "I can do it myself"

• Has a desire to wear "big kid" underwear

• Has the ability to "hold it," or has fewer wet diapers, which likely means their bladder muscles have developed sufficiently.

Differences between potty training (Boys and Girls)

It is not uncommon to hear that potty training girls is easier than boys—and it often happens earlier. That said, every child is different. Your son could be ready at 18 months while your daughter is just beginning to show interest at age 3.

While there are many similarities between potty training for girls and boys—for example, they both respond to potty-training books and videos and both learn sitting down—there are some differences, and parents should be mindful of them.

Girls

• Tend to show interest in toilet training as early as 18 months

• Typically more patient during potty training

• Tend to stick with one reward entirely through toilet training

• Have fewer accidents after learning the initial steps of potty training

Boys

• Tend to take their time, often not ready until age 2

• Typically anxious to hop off toilet and end the lesson

• Tend to get bored with their rewards

• Have more accidents after they seemed to have finished potty training

Potty time supplies

If your child is ready to potty train, take some time to make sure you are armed with the right potty training gear before you proceed, including:

• A potty seat or a seat reducer (or both)

• "Big kid" underwear

• Pants, or other clothing that can be easily pulled on and off

• Charts or potty training rewards (candy, stickers, books, toys) to help keep the little one motivated throughout the process.

Make your child feel like a big kid by bringing them with you to the store to choose a potty, and let them pick out some underwear featuring their favorite characters or color.

Letting your child be involved in the process of choosing these items can heighten their excitement about using the potty.

Tips for potty training

Here are a few more tips for getting your child ready to potty train:

• Teach your child "potty" talk. Use words to express the act of going to the bathroom like "pee," "poop," and "potty."

• Encourage your child to speak up. Ask your child, "Are you going poop in your diaper?" and urge them to tell you when their diaper is wet or soiled.

• Have your child mirror you. Invest in a potty chair, and have your child sit on it while you are using the toilet.

• Watch for telltale signs. Crossing legs, grunting, and squatting are all signs that your child needs to go the bathroom, so if you notice them, urge your child to sit on the potty.

• Be consistent. If a child is being trained during the week with a nanny or at daycare, do not relax the regimen at night or on the weekends. A disruption to the schedule is likely to confuse your toddler and extend the amount of time it takes to train them.

• Set up a schedule. Once your child begins potty training, encourage them to go at set times throughout the day, including when they wake up, after eating, or before nap and bedtime.

• Avoid setting deadlines. Remind yourself that kids potty train at different rates and ages.

• Stay patient. Do not get upset or scold your child when accidents happen, as doing so can set your child back by making potty training a negative experience.

Challenges to potty training

Potty training is a process, so it is important to accept that there will be challenges and hiccups along the way, including:

• Fear of falling into the toilet, or being afraid of the "flushing" sound.

• Having accidents when they are sick, or during a stressful time (new bed, vacation).

• Anxiety about telling other adults they need to go to the bathroom.

• Refusal to go to the bathroom in a public toilet.

• Only wanting to use the potty for peeing, not bowel movements (which can be due to constipation, or lead to it).

• Not being able to hold it overnight—some experts recommended waiting six months after your child is potty trained to ditch nighttime diapers.

The good news is that these are all just minor regressions. Remain calm, and eventually, your child will get back on track toward potty-training success.

CHAPTER 1

FOOD EATEN AND BOWEL MOVEMENT TIMING

A very common situation for potty training children is to learn to urinate in the potty, but then to become hesitant to make a bowel movement there.

Instead of thinking about it as a problem, though, it is better to consider it to be a normal part of potty training.

Before potty training, a child needs to master several important skills, such as being able to sense that they need to poop and then hold it until they reach the toilet; being able to verbalize the need to go to the bathroom to an adult; and being able to undress and redress in order to use the bathroom.

If your child is not ready yet, it is best to wait until they are.

Make pooping on the potty easier

Most children become potty trained sometime between the ages of 18 months and three years. But remember that three years is not a magic age where everyone is potty trained. There are some steps you can take to help your child.

It is estimated that at least 25% of children aren't fully potty trained until they are 3 1/2 or 4 years old.

Provide a footrest

Make sure your child can put their feet on something while sitting on the toilet to poop, as it is difficult to poop when they can not bear down (which requires having your feet on the floor or a step of some kind). This is why kids will often squat in a corner to poop in a diaper, as squatting is a very effective position for getting poop out of the body.

Create a routine

Have your child sit on the toilet at about the same time every day. If there is a time of day that they have typically been pooping in their diaper, choose this time to have them sit on the toilet.

The introduction of food into the stomach sends signals to the colon that make you want to poop (this is called the gastro-colic reflex). So having your child sit on the toilet right after breakfast every day is often a good idea, as the body is primed for pooping then.

Prevent constipation

If your child has bowel movements that are sometimes big, hard and painful to pass, then they may just be afraid to use the potty to have BMs. Constipation often leads to potty training problems.

Make sure your child is drinking plenty of water and has enough fiber in their diet. The American Academy of Pediatrics recommends 7 grams of fiber per day for 2-year-olds and 8 grams for 3-year-olds: their age plus 5. This, along with regular exercise, can help make bowel movements softer and easier to pass. If you have any concerns about constipation in your child, contact your pediatrician for advice.

Reduce stress

Other issues that can lead to potty training issues can include sudden changes at home or daycare, a recent illness, or other stressors. For example, a recent move or new baby in the home can often lead to problems with potty training.3 If this is happening with your child, be patient as they adjust to changes in their life.

Help your child learn to poop on the potty

If constipation is not a problem, and there have not been any recent changes at home, then the following tips may help your child to have regular bowel movements on the potty.

• Continue to let them have bowel movements in a pull-up, but then empty the poop into the potty to show your child where it goes. You can then remind them that "poop goes in the potty."

• Encourage them to have bowel movements in the bathroom, even if that means going in their pull-up. Once they get used to that, then have them sit on the potty in a pull-up when they have to go. Eventually, they may be ready to take it off.

• Offer lots of praise when your child makes progress, whether it is emptying their pull-up in the potty or simply being in the bathroom while they poop in a pull-up. And never scold or punish your child when they don't poop how or where you want them to.

• Read children's storybooks about potty training, such as Everyone Poops or The Princess and the Potty, to help get your child used to the idea of pooping in the potty.

If your child is resistant to all of these methods, continue to give them a pull-up. Let them know that they can tell you when they are ready to start going in the bathroom or on the potty.

Most importantly, do not shame or punish your child for not having bowel movements on the potty. This can quickly turn into a big power struggle, which will make training more difficult.

Speak potty

During potty training sessions, parents often wonder which terms they should use with children. Is language such as bowel movement or urine appropriate, or should parents use more casual terms such as poop and pee?

Language for waste

Whether to use the clinically correct terms for waste is a highly personal decision and frequently involves one's own family history. People with parents who said "pee" and "poop" will likely use these terms with their children.

There is nothing wrong with either style. You won't be doing your child any injustice or harm by using childish words to describe these things. They are a child, after all, and unless you plan to hide them away, they will eventually learn both the correct terms and some slang that might make you cringe.

Language for body parts

When talking about parts of the body, however, doctors strongly recommend using proper anatomical names. Just as you would not call an elbow or an eye a silly name, you should not call a penis a "wee wee."

Knowing the correct names for private parts can help protect children from sexual abuse and ensure that they get proper medical care. Helping your child learn about all the parts of their body also promotes a positive body image.

Use the potty language of child care

In her book The Girlfriend's Guide to Toddlers, Vicki Iovine sums it up nicely: "What good is it to teach your child to ask his daycare provider whether he/she can go to the bathroom to void when all the other kids are being told it is time to go potty? It cannot help but be useful for potty trainees to share a common potty language."

Ask your child care provider the words used at preschool and incorporate that language into your home repertoire as well.

Avoid shaming

Children may be confused if you completely eliminate or discourage certain words or add negative emotion to words. This is why a penis should be called a penis, and a vagina a vagina.

Do you find it embarrassing or feel some sense of shame over these words even though they are not curse words and would be appropriate to use in public? This attitude can easily be conveyed to your child, especially if you and your spouse argue about it or you admonish or correct them in front of your child when they use these words.

Parents teach children to be embarrassed by or ashamed of their genitalia by the parent's own words and actions towards them. A parent's reluctance or unwillingness to use the correct terms sends a message to the child that this is not a subject the parent wants to discuss.

You want your child to feel comfortable talking about all aspects of using the bathroom with you. If they are experiencing pain or itching, for example, you need to know about it; your child may need medical care, and you'll both need to tell the doctor what is going on.

Potty language should be rated G

If the words you or your spouse are using would not be used around a group of your peers (meaning other parents of toddlers), then you should definitely talk to your partner about using more appropriate terms.

There is nothing cute or developmentally appropriate about teaching a toddler to swear. And it's nearly impossible to teach a toddler that it is fine to say one word at home but not to use that same word at preschool or a friend's house.

If your family has been using words that would carry an R-rating, stop immediately and do your best to ignore the behavior in your toddler. It can be tempting to make a big deal about banning the words or creating a scary label but this almost always makes the problem worse and gives the offending word more allure to your toddler. Modeling the appropriate language instead will go a long way toward changing the behavior.

Introduce to toilet

If you have the time and patience and want to avoid diapers as much as possible, you can start watching your child for patterns and cues that allow potty training to begin when your child is just a baby. Here is how to get started with infant potty training, also known as elimination communication.

Infant potty training

In other cultures, some parents never use disposable diapers. Even the cloth diapers that we are familiar with aren't used at all. Babies are wrapped in thin strips of cloth, allowed to be naked and worn by their mothers or siblings in slings or dressed in light clothing without many fasteners. Placing a child on the potty or holding him while he goes potty somewhere, then, is not the ordeal that it would be in the United States or other countries where babies wear diapers, diaper covers and layers of clothing over that.

In these same cultures, mothers, siblings, and other caregivers spend a lot of time in very close proximity to their babies. A mother is able to recognize certain cues that the baby gives when he needs to use the bathroom.

In addition, parents and caregivers also know the child's routines and patterns of eating, sleeping and going to the bathroom.

As a result, potty training beginning as early as birth is practiced. In the United States, this is known as infant potty training or elimination communication. In other countries, it is seen as the natural way children learn to use the bathroom.

For most of us, the norm is to immediately wrap a diaper around a baby's bottom and then wait passively until he poops or pees so we can clean up the mess. Our active role takes place after the event. In cultures where babies do not wear diapers, a caregiver's active role takes place before and during the event.

Getting started

Some proponents believe that there is an optimal window for starting the infant potty training between birth and about 6 months. Others have experienced success starting later.

The key to remember is that you, the parent, will be responsible for recognizing when your child needs to use the bathroom before he goes. You will also be responsible for taking him and putting him on the potty each time.

If you go into infant potty training with that in mind, then you have got your expectations set correctly. If, however, you feel that your child should be the one to let you know or should possess some sort of awareness at this early age, your expectations are unrealistic and you should not attempt this process. Awareness on your child's part is very gradual, as is his participation.

Now that you have got the right mindset, you will need to get physically prepared. To prepare your child's environment, you will just need to buy cloth diapers, very small underwear (doll underwear can work) or just dress your child in his clothes without anything on underneath. Some parents prefer to let their child be naked and that is fine, too, as long as he/she is warm enough.

Be ready for accidents to happen. It will take some time to recognize the signs and you will make mistakes at first.

That is alright. Another way to look at it is that if you wait until your child is a toddler, you will be experiencing accidents, too, only they are much bigger than a baby's accidents.

Some parents may be tempted to use disposable diapers and while that is up to you, it can hinder the process and set you up for failure. The success of this method depends on you quickly recognizing patterns and learning your child's toileting habits.

Disposable diapers can impair your ability to recognize when your child has just wet or soiled himself and delay your awareness. Some disposable diapers are so good at what they do, it is hard to even tell if they are wet when your child has only gone a small amount.

Purchase waterproof pads to go in your child's sleeping area and places where your child may be like car seats, underneath a blanket on the floor or on your lap. A sling is also a wonderful tool for infant potty training. You will need to observe your baby for signs all the time, and there's no better way to do that than by wearing him close to your body. In addition, buy one of the books on the topic that explain the process in depth and have information about troubleshooting problems that could arise.

Purchasing a potty chair is optional. Some parents prefer to use something smaller, while for others, one of the major points of this method is not having to buy or consume all the stuff of potty training. Using the toilet is completely fine. Just watch out for splashing water. If you know it's your child's poop time, a wad of toilet paper placed in the bowl first can help alleviate that issue.

After you have got the environment ready, you are ready to start observing your child and watching for the following signs which indicate he/she is about to urinate or have a bowel movement:

- Crying or fussiness just before going

- Grunting

- Squinting

- Red face

- Kicking legs or flailing arms

- Squirming

- Muscle tension, especially in the abdomen

- Reaching for or touching the genital area

While your child is actively urinating or having a bowel movement, you may notice:

- Active pushing

- Contraction of the abdomen

- A faraway look

- He/she stops nursing briefly and then resumes

- He/she stops other activities and then resumes

- Reaching for or touching the genital area.

Your child may also have his/her own unique signs and body language. Over time as you watch your baby carefully, you will begin to pick up on these. Babies sometimes very early on develop a special sound to indicate they would like to nurse, and likewise, he/she may develop a special sound to indicate his/her potty needs. You can encourage this by making the same sounds yourself while he/she is going. Some parents like to make a soft sound while the baby is urinating or just hum.

Another name for infant potty training is elimination communication. So, think of it as a mutual exchange between you and your child. He/she will begin to pick up on your signs, just as you are picking up on his/hers.

In addition to watching for and learning your child's signs, you will want to get to know his routine (which you can control to some degree by determining bedtimes, bathtimes, playtimes and feeding times) and his/her body's timing. How long is it after he/she eats before he/she is ready to have a bowel movement? Does he/she urinate first thing in the morning? It helps to write these times down while you are looking for patterns and getting to know how the child operates.

When your child is ready to use the potty or even if it is just close to time, you just securely hold him/her over it and let him/her go. Clean any residue with toilet paper and/or wipes afterward. Some children start to recognize where they are and what they are supposed to do there early in the process so even if they are not completely ready, a couple of minutes after you begin holding them over the potty, they're ready to use it.

Of course, for safety reasons, never try to prop your child on a toilet or potty chair at this age and do not ever leave him unattended. This is an active process that involves parent and child interacting closely, carefully and constantly.

When does infant potty training end?

Eventually, your child will become more aware of not only the urges and sensations associated with using the bathroom but also the routine you have already in place. Once he starts walking, you can guide him to the potty and when he's able to follow verbal commands, you can simply tell him to go potty. There will be a period of time where it is still you who shoulders the responsibility of knowing when it is time to go, but slowly you will see your child's potty independence emerge. Play it by ear and make sure you are backing off sometimes so that your child can step up to the task.

One of the great bonuses of this method is that many of the issues parents face who begin potty training their children later are removed. Your child will already be used to the bathroom environment, won't be afraid to use a potty and won't need to be introduced to underwear, for example. This can lead to earlier independence in some cases.

Practice

The most important thing to remember is that potty training is a process and your child will have accidents, but stick to this method and your child will be using the potty consistently in just three days.

Is your child ready? Preparing for infant potty training

Before deciding to take the leap and potty train, you should get your child familiar with using the toilet. Let your child come with you to the bathroom and show him what big boys and girls do.

Most kids are excited to learn about bathroom etiquette. Show them how the toilet flushing works and how to wash their hands. Look for signs of readiness and excitement, such as your child telling you when he has to pee or poop; asking you to use the potty; feeling bothered by a dirty diaper.

Does your child seem excited to use the potty? The three-day method will only work if your child is on board.

Choose the weekend

You will need three days in a row where you are home with your child. For working parents, this method works best over a three day weekend or a time when you can take off a day of work to add on to a regular Saturday/Sunday.

You will be inside for most of the weekend so it important to mentally prepare yourself to spend lots of time with your child. Have fun with them! If you cannot block out three days, on the final day, discuss what you have been doing with your childcare provider and ask them to continue the process.

Stock up

Once your child is showing signs of readiness, take them to a store and pick out underwear together. Purchasing underwear with their favorite characters is a fun way to get them excited about wearing big boy or big girl underwear.

Also, since you will be spending a lot of time at home, you may want to think about some at-home projects in advance. This may be art supplies, a movie, games, cooking, baking or anything else that will keep you and your child entertained.

Before the long weekend

One week in advance, let your child know that it is time to say "goodbye" to diapers. Depending on what your family decides, this could be a full goodbye or a partial goodbye where diapers or pull-ups will be used during nap and bedtime. Once you start training, underwear will be worn at all times unless your child is sleeping.

If you are doing a full goodbye to diapers, you can count the remaining diapers with the child and explain that when they are gone there are no more. You can still make sure only one diaper is left before bedtime the night before you begin toilet training.

Share the process with your spouse and other caregivers, such as babysitters, nannies, and relatives. Take shifts (especially if there is an older sibling) or stay together and support each other during the process.

It is important that all adults are involved in the process and that using the toilet does not become something that is done only with one adult in the family. By sharing the responsibility, your child learns that they must use the toilet with everyone, not just in certain situations or with specific adults.

Day 1

Right when your child wakes up, change their out of the diaper. Let your child spend at least the first day bare-bottomed. Without a diaper or underpants on your child will be more likely to recognize the need to use the toilet.

You may choose to put a little potty in the living room for easy access.

This is a personal choice as some people may want to keep all bathroom activities in the bathroom. Give your child a big glass of water, juice, or milk so they have to pee frequently. Have a constant sippy cup near your child's reach. Give your child a lot of fluid and watch intently for signs that your child is about to pee or poop.

When you notice the sign, take your child to the bathroom immediately to use the toilet. Ask them if they have to go every 20 minutes. You may want to set an audible 20-minute timer so your child knows that when the timer goes off it is time to try to use the toilet. Make sure to have your child wash hands after each attempt to instill healthy habits.

If your child does not want to try, you could say we are going to try "after you are done playing with your trains" or if your kids know numbers, you could say "we are going to try when the clock says "10:30." Have your child attempt to use the toilet at every transition, after cleaning up a toy/material, before snack or lunch, and before and after nap and bedtime. This will become part of their daily routine.

Use emotionally neutral, behavioral observations regarding your child's progress. "You peed in the toilet, that is where pee belongs!" or "you peed on the floor, help me clean it up."

You know your child best. Some children respond well to an exciting celebration of success while others become uncomfortable with the attention. Some children respond well to rewards so if your child is motivated by stickers or small treats, you may decide to do a reward chart to encourage potty training.

Day 2 and Day 3

Your process for day 2 and 3 is essentially the same as day 1. Some people stay inside on all 3 days to solidify the process. Other people choose to venture outside for short activities on the afternoon of day 2 and day 3.

If you go outside, go to a playground or do an activity that is close by and always remember to bring a small portable potty with you in case your child refuses to use the public restroom, as some kids do. Expect accidents. When they happen, just change the underwear and don't make a big deal. Simply say, "we pee and poop in the potty."

Toilet training tips

• Have your child use the toilet before leaving home and immediately upon arriving at their destination.

• Bring multiple changes of clothing and underwear when you go out.

• Tell your teachers, daycare providers, nannies, and babysitters your child's signs when he or she needs to use the potty and what language you use at home so they can be consistent with your preferences (pee, poop, toilet, potty, doo doo, BM, tinkle, etc).

• Being without a diaper is a new sensation and it may feel uncomfortable or scary for some children. Remain calm and reassuring as you support your child during this process. Research has shown that a negative reaction or punishment after an accident can create a negative association with toileting and can hinder progress, so to remain calm after an accident and hide any frustration from the child.

• Believe in the process. It is very easy to get discouraged on day 2 when your child is having accidents, but once you make it to day 3 and beyond, your child will show you that he or she understands what it means to be potty trained.

Forsake diapers

Toilet training is hard—especially when your child keeps insisting on a diaper. No wonder, few concerns generate as much angst and self-doubt among parents as teaching this routine, daily business.

It seems so simple. Once your child can sense they need to go to the bathroom, then they can and will start using the toilet rather than diapers. Right? Well, like those in the trenches know, it is rarely that easy.

Similar to the wealth of advice and strategies on handling the familiar challenges of how to get them to go to (and stay in) bed (tear-free) and eat their peas (without spitting them out), there are enough theories on the best potty training methods to make your head spin. This gets even trickier when you are in the midst of teaching your child to use the bathroom but they keep insisting on a diaper instead.

What you need is to get on the same team. Sorting through the pros and cons of all the different approaches to eradicating the diaper is challenging at best. Try the below suggestions so you can get back to closely monitoring whether those wiggles mean somebody needs to find a potty.

Make sure your child is ready

You will have a good sense that your child Is developmentally able to work toward this skill when they start regularly showing the typical signs. Look out for the following indicators of readiness:

• Brings you a diaper to go in it or to change into after soiling a diaper.

• Can follow a simple series of instructions.

- Dislikes the sensation of wet or messy diapers.

- Exhibits increasing independence, as in wanting to be "a big kid" and "do it by myself."

- Is interested in "big kid pants."

- Is willing to try.

- Knows when they need to go (at least some of the time).

- Shows an interest in using the toilet

Why kids resist giving up diapers

It is important to note that even if your child exhibits signs of readiness, they still may cling to the diaper. Frustrating as this can be (for child and parent alike), know it is very common and also likely not intended as defiance.

Giving up the diaper, like any rite of passage while growing up, could feel genuinely upsetting—they are called "growing pains" for a reason.

Change is hard for all of us, and it is normal to stick to the comfort of our routines and what is known. To that end, it is key to capitalize on when your child no longer can tolerate a wet or dirty diaper (as in no longer finds the diaper comfortable)—and understand that you may need to push your little one a little bit out of their comfort zone to help them learn this vital skill.

Another reason a child might prefer a diaper is a worry of disappointing you or themselves with accidents. Therefore, it is helpful (and good for a child's self-esteem) to focus on the successes.

Praise and celebrate any positive steps, from keeping a diaper dry to alerting you right away when they did not make it in time, or even just a willingness to try. Use any mishaps (in most cases, there will be many) along the way as teaching moments and avoid scolding, shaming, or punishments.

Stubbornness may also play a part—and that is OK. Young children learn by testing boundaries and build independence by making their own decisions.

Power struggles are par for the course when we seek to implement new routines, teach new skills, or alter our expectations. Adapting to letting go of diapers is no different.

Guide your child to success

Loving patience combined with holding firm to your objectives tends to work wonders. Aim to defuse rather than fan any power plays that pop-up. Equally important is to listen to your child.

Have empathy for their concerns and the fact that taking this leap towards bathroom independence is a big deal. It might even feel scary or sad.

They might resist because they still want to be your "baby." They may really like the design imprinted on their diapers (a problem solved by providing equally enticing big kid pants). Or, they might just like getting a rise out of you—and your attention.

But you might not find out why unless you take the time to observe and listen. Once they feel heard and their concerns are aired, you'll likely see greater compliance with your potty training plan.

Diapers and potty training

If you believe your child's reliance on diapers is getting in the way of toilet training, you may consider making them off-limits or limiting their use. For instance, you could choose to completely stop providing diapers.

This approach is best if you are following a fast and intensive potty training method where you spend several days focused exclusively on using the bathroom. Or, you might simply set aside designated times when your child can use them, such as during naps and/or outings, as well as prescribing times when your child will go without them.

Consistency in your policy is important, as well as creating a reliable toileting routine so your child knows what to expect and what your expectations are for them as well. Also, be sure to let your child know it is OK if they are a little upset about having to let go of using diapers.

You may want to work some flexibility into your plan, such as allowing an insisted upon diaper when your child is especially tired, not feeling well, or you have company over and cannot give the potty training efforts your full attention. However, for the most part, holding firm in a kind, reassuring, encouraging way—even in the face of a tantrum or two—will send the message to your child that they are, in fact, ready to master this skill.

Consistency and follow-through are key. If you say, "No more diapers!" mean it. If you hand your child a diaper every time they want one, don't be surprised if they keep insisting on using them.

Out of sight, out of mind

For those kids who are especially attached to their diapers, it may be helpful to remove diapers from any place your child can see or get them. If you intend to go cold turkey, then it may ease the transition for your child if diapers aren't a visible temptation or reminder.

If you plan to move away from diapers more gradually, only bring them out at times (if using them at all) that their use is part of your potty training agenda, such as at bedtime or for a long car ride. If you are keeping the diapers on hand, be sure to put them in a place that is truly out of reach and out of sight like a cabinet with a safety lock.

Remember your reaction to your child's demands for diapers will be an essential factor in whether this works.

When your child asks (or wails) for a diaper when you want them to use the potty, try very calmly and firmly directing them to use the potty. Remind them that diapers are for bedtime only (or whatever your policy is).

Most importantly, avoid giving in to tears or tantrums. Instead, find another way to help your child feel supported. Soon enough, once they realize that you mean business, your little one will recognize it is time to try the potty.

That said, it is worth considering if your child's persistent demands for diapers may mean they just aren't quite ready. If you are not sure, review the readiness cues. If the signs do not seem to be there quite yet, it might be worth holding off on your efforts for a month or two.

Remember, there is no one right time. Forcing the issue may end up delaying success. Giving your child some extra time and space may even result in a faster, more positive potty training experience when you are both ready to try again.

Stay calm and encouraging

It is natural for you both to get worked up at times during this race to the potty but be attuned to the fact that your child will respond to a calm, self-disciplined attitude much better than to an annoyed one.

When your child has an inevitable accident, do not punish them or react with exasperation. Simply tell them that it's time to get cleaned up and help them with the cleanup steps. Use phrases like, "Good try," "Potty training is hard work" and "You really tried hard, I bet next time make it to the potty."

Instill self-confidence and pride in your child to convey that you believe in their future success.

While most kids do fine going back and forth between a diaper or disposable training pants at night and underwear during the day, some do not.

For those kids, having a diaper sometimes is confusing and may cause them to dig in and avoid daytime potty training.

In these cases, it may work better to go with thick training pants, fewer fluids in the evening hours, and a protective covering on the bed. The inconvenience of a wet bed now and then will be made up for with a less confused child, no mixed messages about where it is OK to go to the bathroom, and potty training success during the day.

CHAPTER 2

PLAY WITH AND CELEBRATE BABY FOR POTTYING

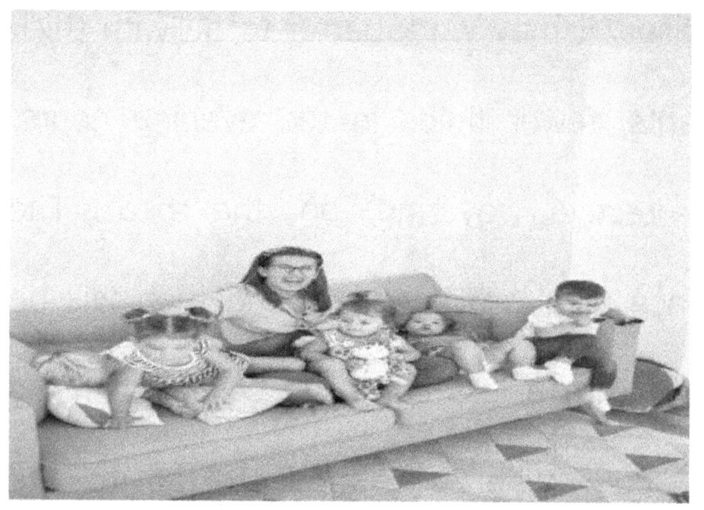

Preschool-age children are learning a lot. From potty training to controlling their temper, they are discovering what is expected of them and trying to do their best. Parents can encourage good behavior by setting up a reward system that is sure to get their attention.

Why is a reward system important for preschoolers?

Here is the thing about preschoolers. They like to do things their own way on their own time. So when you want to encourage a new behavior — potty training, doing simple chores, or something of the like — a great way to do it is to set up a reward system.

A positive form of discipline, a reward system for children does not have to be complicated. It can be as simple as stickers on a chart or buttons or beans in a jar. Whatever method you choose, the object is to keep track of good behavior so your child will continue acting that way in the future.

Setting up a reward system for your children

1. Explain the concept to your preschooler. Before you start, talk to your preschooler about what it is you would like him/her to strive for.

In my friend's house, it was getting her three-year-old to pull up his own pants after he went to the bathroom. For others, it may be how many days she can go without a temper tantrum or for every meal she is able to clear her plate.

Whatever the behavior, explain to your preschooler what you are looking for and what the ground rules are.

2. Set ground rules. In our case, my son could earn two stickers each time he went to the bathroom — one for pulling up his underpants and one for pulling up his pants or shorts. He had to pull them all the way up in order to earn his prize.

Talk about what it is you want your preschooler to do and what she needs to do to succeed. Some parents like to offer a grand prize — fill up the bean jar or earn 25 stickers and the child gets an additional reward.

When setting up ground rules, do whatever works best for your family.

3. Create a reward system. Get your preschooler in on the process.

Gather up posterboard or cardboard, a jar, or whatever you are using, as well as markers and stickers and let your preschooler decorate. If you are making a chart, make sure the tallying method is clear so it is easy to keep track of any rewards your child earns.

4. Try to focus on one or two behaviors at a time. You may have a litany of things you want your preschooler to work on, but it is a good idea to tackle only one at any given time.

If you are potty training and working on sticking to a bedtime routine, consider adding chores to your preschooler's schedule on the back burner.

Having too many "to-do's" on your preschooler's list can be confusing (for you and the child). It can also lead to many reward charts decorating your walls (although you might save money on the wallpaper).

5. Payout perks promptly. Here is the key to a successful reward system — it must be immediate.

Whether you choose to use a sticker chart or beans in a jar, make sure as soon as your child does the target behavior those stickers or beans are in hand and ready to go. When they go on the potty or get through a meal without a temper tantrum they can be duly recorded.

Most preschoolers have no real sense of time yet, so by offering the sticker up right away, you are confirming their good behavior and encouraging them to do it again.

6. Be consistent. In the same vein as being prompt, you need to make sure you are consistent in handing out awards. And do not give one out if your child has not done the targeted behavior.

Caregivers' role

Caregivers who see your child every day are often the first to notice signs that your toddler is ready to potty train. To successfully potty train in partnership with your daycare or an experienced nanny or sitter, communication is crucial.

For working parents, it is important to talk to caregivers about your potty training expectations and plans. An experienced nanny or sitter might be able to provide guidance and even lead the way on potty training. Whatever the case may be, it is important that everyone commits to the same potty training process.

Nap and nighttime

Whether or not to put a diaper on during nap and nighttime during three-day potty training is a personal decision. Some believe it is easier to potty train completely for daytime, naps, and nighttime; others train in stages.

Your children can often be helpful in decision making, too.

Although worrisome, bedwetting is a perfectly normal behavior for preschool-aged children who have just been potty trained—perhaps as often as a three or four times a week.

Children (preschoolers and older) may wet their bed when they are under stress or because there is another underlying medical or emotional cause.

Steps to get past bedwetting

There are some steps you can take as a parent to support your child and prevent bet wetting. They include:

• Put a limit on the number of drinks your child has after a certain point in the evening. For example, you let them have one last drink about an hour before bedtime.

• Make sure your child goes to the bathroom before they go to bed.

• If your child falls asleep (and back to sleep) easily, wake them up a little later to go to the potty again before you or your partner goes to bed.

• Without putting any pressure on your child, have a chat with them at bedtime about why staying dry through the night is important. Make sure your child knows that it is OK to get up and go to the bathroom during the night if they need to.

The most important thing is that your child knows bedwetting is not their fault. Children under the age of seven do not yet have the bladder capacity to stay dry all night. They are also still learning to recognize bodily signals telling them they need to use the bathroom.

The expression, "That is why we call it an accident and not an on purpose" totally fits the bill here. Do not make your child feel guilty for bedwetting—chances are they already feel bad enough as it is. Instead, let your child know that you are there to support and help them.

Potty training tricks

Employing the methods that you used to initially potty train your preschooler can also help curb bedwetting.

For example, a sticker chart is a great way to positively reinforce dry nights. Reward your child once they've collected a set number—say, a whole week without wetting the bed.

If your child does have a bedwetting accident, continue the reason. If your child starts wetting the bed after being dry all night for six months, consider what is going on in their life.

Is there a new sibling in the house? Are you in the middle of a divorce? Has the child lost a close family member? Stress, especially life-changing occurrences can cause any child to wet the bed.

If this happens, reassure your child that everything is going to be OK and that you will work on it together. However, if the nighttime accidents are frequent or increasing—especially if they aren't tied to a specific stressor—there may be another cause.

If your child turns six years old and they are still wetting the bed twice a week or more for longer than week, talk to your pediatrician. Your child's doctor can do a thorough exam and determine if your child's bedwetting has a medical cause that needs to be treated.

Accidents

Potty training can be a trying experience for both the child and the parents. Success does not usually come without accidents—and likely some tears or other setbacks—along the way. Learning to use the toilet is not a one-size-fits-all endeavor. Regardless of how your potty training experience is going, it is important to make sure your child feels supported and that you communicate a positive attitude while they work to master this new skill.

While positivity is key, there are some definite "don'ts" you need to know—and avoid falling into. Below are some of the most common well-intentioned but ultimately counterproductive traps to steer clear of while potty training your child.

➢ Do not force the issue

Make sure that your child is developmentally ready to use the potty before you start training. Typical signs of readiness include a child being able to communicate their needs, showing an interest in bathroom independence, and the ability to handle the physical requirements, such as dressing themselves, feeling when they "need to go" and following a series of simple steps. If you suspect your child may not be ready, it's advisable to give them a few more weeks or months before trying again.

If your child refuses to go, forcing them to go and sit on the potty will likely create a negatively charged atmosphere and can ultimately lead to more resistance. This can produce negative associations with using the bathroom that can be hard to undo and may cause your child to withhold urinating or voiding, which can be harmful.

Always aim to offer encouragement and support. If the process becomes a battle, even if your child otherwise seems "ready" you might consider putting on the brakes. You will get the best success (with potty training and your relationship) if both of you are enthusiastic about this "big kid" step.

Try to approach this time of learning much the same as you did with other milestones like sitting up, walking, and talking. Honor that while almost all kids get there, some take a little more time and patience to master these skills.

> Do not start potty training during a time of stress

Even good stress is bad stress when it comes to potty training. Marriages, new babies, holidays, visitors, and vacations can be unsettling for your child—similar to the challenges of coping with a divorce, death, or a move to a new home.

If anything big and new is on the horizon in your lives, reconsider potty training right now. Wait until life settles down and the normal flow of activity resumes. This creates security for your child and helps them place toileting easily alongside other normal routines. Plus, you will have more attention and positive energy to put towards helping your child transition out of diapers.

➢ Do not set deadlines

More often than not, young children do not work well under deadlines and they do not have the same concept of time as adults do. Be realistic with your potty training expectations. Or, better yet, throw them out the window altogether. Know that kids potty train at different rates and ages. Some kids learn before 18 months, but many take a year to a few years more until they are ready. Some do not master the skill until just before kindergarten. While a few kids do toilet train rapidly, for many, it is a much longer process.

Programs that promise that your child will be potty trained in three days, one day or even 100 days aren't taking your child's individuality into account. Each child has a unique temperament and developmental schedule, and they bring different skills to the table, so there is no true one-size-fits-all method out there.

Programs that operate under a time schedule often suggest punitive measures, are inflexible or are actually training the parents (as in having you monitor your child's every grimace or race your child to the bathroom every 10 minutes) instead of the child. This sets many parents and children who don't meet the deadline up for a feeling of failure and lots of unhealthy stress.

In addition, they may not take into consideration the many different lifestyles families have, which include parents who work, families with many children, children with special needs, multiples, and parents who share custody. Make sure any method you use is flexible and meets the needs of everyone involved. Most importantly, choose a potty training method the helps your child feel good about the process, whether it takes a few days or many months.

> ➢ Do not treat accidents like a big deal

One of the cornerstones of positive and effective potty training models is to remember that "it is just a normal part of life." Reinforce to your child that going to the bathroom—and the occasional accident—is natural and nothing to feel badly about.

Accidents happen, and when they do, we learn from them as part of the expected process.

Overemphasizing accidents can actually reinforce mishaps or amplify feelings of shame, leading to more accidents. So, when they occur, keep the tone even and matter-of-fact, or even silly. Enlist your child in clean-up activity and move on to the next opportunity to use the potty.

> Do not use clothes that are difficult to manage

Ask any childcare teacher who is in charge of a group of potty trainees and they will tell you just how difficult it can be for little arms and hands to manipulate complicated buttons, snaps, zippers, pants, overalls, multiple layers, and other unwieldy clothing when the urge to pee or poop is looming.

Make it as easy as possible for your child. Use your child's motor skills as a gauge when choosing clothes during potty training. Simple elastic waist pants, shorts, or skirts are ideal for most.

Shy away from overalls unless your child is adept at removing them and putting them back on. The same is true for suspenders, belts, tights, one-piece shirts that snap at the crotch, and anything with lots of zippers, snaps, buttons, or other fasteners that might be a challenge for your child to manage quickly and independently.

When at home, consider letting your child run around in just underwear or in the nude if you are comfortable with it. After all, it is the ultimate potty training outfit. Many parents advocate for this approach, as it works well to let our child know right away if they need to go (or just missed getting) to the bathroom.

Since winter in colder climates is a time of layers, bundling, and heavy coats, most experts and parents agree that it may not the optimal time to start potty training. When potty training in the summer, kids wearing swim trunks or two-piece swimsuits have it made. Kids in one-piece suits will face a bigger challenge pulling them off (especially when wet). Opting for swim outfits with a separate bottom will make it easier to remove as needed.

➢ Do not give in to external pressures

External pressures (in terms of how and when to potty train and how quickly results should come) can arrive from many sources: Grandparents, other parents at the playgroup, preschool administrators, teachers, and partners. Keep in mind that while others may be full of wisdom about childrearing, some advice just may not resonate for you or won't work best for you and your child. Go with your own instincts and rely on the knowledge you have about your child's readiness and the approaches that make you (and your child) the most comfortable.

Whether intentioned or not, it is easy to end up feeling judged, less than, or in competition with other parents around the timetables our kids meet various skills. Remember that these are skills that the vast majority of children will learn—they all just learn at different times, at their own pace. Resist getting caught up in worrying about who potty trained first or quickest or easiest. Ultimately, it does not really matter and can just end up making you feel stressed or just plain bad.

➢ Do not blindly follow school timetables

Schools that require your child to be potty trained by a certain age may do so simply to meet licensing standards or avoid inconvenience. Licensing standards require that any room with a child in diapers be equipped with a diaper changing table and a sink as well as other supplies. If the sink must have hot water at a temperature that differs from that of the sink available to children, this can mean that the school must run new plumbing from a separate hot water heater.

Schools may not want to deal with the hassle of equipping a room, or they may not want to spend the money. Think about it this way, if the school is already setting an arbitrary deadline for toileting skills and not taking into account the individual needs of each child, what other areas will they apply this thinking to as well? If this is the reality at your school and you have options, it may be worth considering whether it is the right school for you or your child.

> ➤ Do not expect night time training right away

Generally speaking, urinary control comes before control of bowel movements and dry nights come well behind both. It is completely normal for bed-wetting (or enuresis) to occur in children until they are 4 years old or older.

According to the American Academy of Pediatrics (AAP), about 20% of 5-year-olds and up to 10% of 7-year-olds experience bed-wetting. For many children, bladder control at night comes years later and bed-wetting does not necessarily signify any medical problem. Know that many healthy kids out there use pull-ups or wet the bed occasionally well into elementary school, but do not hesitate to speak to your child's pediatrician if you are concerned. The vast majority grow out of this naturally as their body develops greater urinary control—it just takes time.

The AAP lists two main factors: Your child's bladder may not yet have developed the ability to hold urine the whole night and/or they have not learned to recognize when they have to go, to wake up, make it to the toilet, and use it. For a child who is asleep, that's a four-step process. Some kids are such deep sleepers that they just do not wake up before it is too late.

Trusting that your child will get there eventually and not putting too much emphasis on it as a "problem" lets your child know that what they are experiencing is normal and nothing to be ashamed about, which in turn can help speed along the process.

> ➢ Do not discount your child's fears or attachments

Children can develop fears during potty training, and they are as large to them as fears adults may have. Kids can also get scared of something you would never think of as an adult. The important thing is to honor and care for their feelings.

Children may not understand the mechanics of the toilet and that loud flushing sound in that small space can be frightening. If a child experiences even one slip off the toilet seat and their bottom touch water, it could set them back to square one or even require a potty training hiatus. Some children have a hard time dealing with watching their poop disappear down the drain as if it were as much a part of them as an arm or a leg.

Treat these fears with sensitivity. Discuss the fear without invalidating it or making your child feel as if their feelings are unimportant. Some children may need help expressing their concerns and coping with their feelings, so offer them the vocabulary that seems appropriate.

The same is true of attachments children may exhibit during this time. Diapers may represent a feeling of security or "special" babyhood. It is a time when parents are intimate with their children and are taking care of their needs, and letting go of that takes some children more time.

This does not mean you need to abandon training or let your child choose to go back and forth between wearing diapers and training whenever they want, but it does mean making sure they are ready to take that step of independence. If your child seems to want to cling to diapers, suggest that it is potty time and offer that afterward (whether they have used the potty or not) they can have a story on your lap, some tickle-time, or another special activity. It may not be the diaper your child missing but rather the closeness with you. It can be cold and lonely in the bathroom, after all.

➤ Keep moving regardless

It is not unusual for younger children to have setbacks with potty training. In fact, many children aren't fully toilet trained by age three, especially for bowel movements. Still, potty training regression is frustrating for parents. Remember that it is normal, common and temporary.

Causes of potty training regression

Sometimes, regression is simply due to distraction, or an unwillingness to give up a toy or activity. Your child might be waiting until the last minute to go and does not make it to the bathroom in time. Many children do not want to take a break from playing to go to the bathroom.

- **Stress and other emotional setbacks**

Stress is a common cause of regressions in potty training. Changes like starting school or changing classrooms or teachers could trigger a regression. Changes at home, such as a new baby, a new home, or a divorce, can also commonly cause regressions. Or if your child had an accident at school or somewhere else in public and felt shamed, they might regress in their potty progress.

- **Constipation and other physical issues**

If your child seems constipated and is having large, hard, or very firm bowel movements, then you may need to address that problem before working on potty training again. Children with constipation can have painful bowel movements that make them afraid to go on the potty or toilet.

If untreated, these children can begin to hold their bowel movements for so long that they eventually cannot tell when they have to go and have stooling accidents. This is called encopresis and is often confused with potty training refusal.

Urinary tract infections or intestinal bugs may also scare a child away from the potty for a time.

What to do about potty training regression

If it is a medical issue, get advice from your pediatrician. Otherwise, if your child is distracted or working through another change, such as a new sibling, these steps may help.

- **Provide a regular schedule**

Set up a simple potty schedule, or remind your child to go every 2 or 3 hours. Try having them sit on the potty for 4 to 5 minutes when they wake up and after meals. Those are times when most children are likely to have a bowel movement. Offer praise and extra attention simply for trying.

This is likely not a time to go back to diapers or pull-ups. Avoid this along with anything else that makes your child feel ashamed for having accidents.

- **Keep cool when accidents happen**

Treat accidents lightly. That means cleaning them up in a calm, matter-of-fact way, without punishment. As Vicki Lansky says in her book titled *Toilet Training: A Practical Guide to Daytime and Nighttime Training*, do not overreact to accidents.

You want to be careful that you do not reinforce this behavior, and negative attention will do that. You also want to avoid power struggles.

- **Read and reward**

A reward chart for the days when your child does not have an accident can be helpful, as you can be reading some of the potty training books for children. Keep reminding your child (and yourself) that they can do this. Eventually, they will!